Certified Mental Health Technician

Study Guide

Author By Natasha Cossom BHSC, RMA (AMT)
Co-Author X.R. Newman MSHI, BSHCA, CPI, AHI

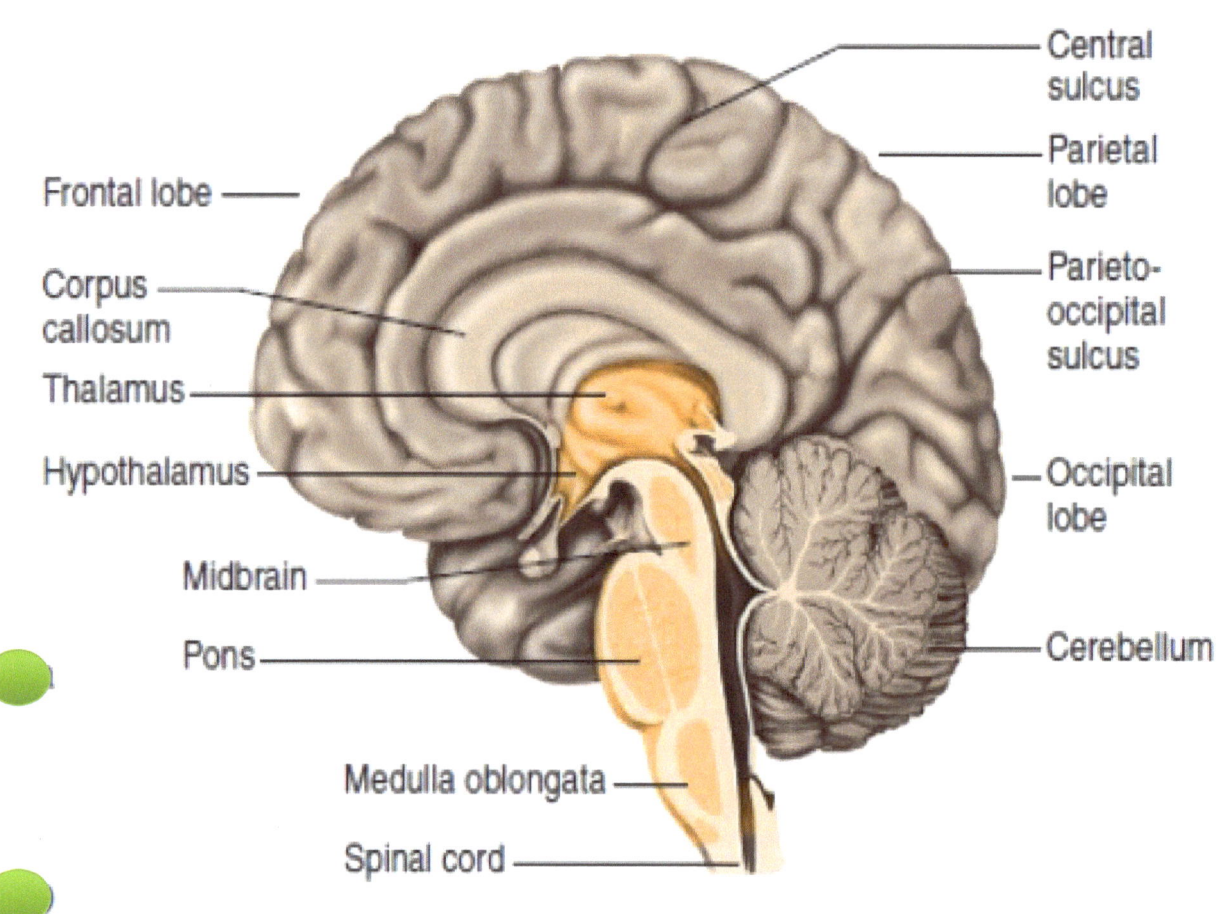

Frontal lobe ——

Corpus callosum ——

Thalamus ——

Hypothalamus ——

Midbrain ——

Pons ——

Medulla oblongata ——

Spinal cord ——

Central sulcus

Parietal lobe

Parieto-occipital sulcus

Occipital lobe

Cerebellum

Certified Mental Health Technician

Certified Mental Health Technician/ Psychiatric Technician

Introduction

Mental Health Technicians, also called psychiatric aides, work with mentally retarded, emotionally disturbed, or psychiatric patients under the supervision of a psychiatrist, psychologist, registered nurse or social worker. They participate in the development and implementation of therapeutic treatment plans for emotionally disabled patients. Treatment plans include recreational, occupational and readjustment activities. The technician participates in group therapy with patients and their families, refers patients to community agencies, and visits patients after their release from an institution. The mental health technician attends to patients' physical needs and well-being. This exam does not credential you to be a mental health therapist, or for the private practice of mental health counseling.

Practice settings

Mental Health Technicians have special training in two areas that have a tremendous unmet need -- treatment programs for the mentally ill and developmentally disabled. Mental health technicians work in private and public mental health hospitals or on the psychiatric wards of general hospitals, mental health clinics, schools for the mentally retarded, drug and alcohol rehabilitation clinics, nursing homes, community agencies and human services programs. In a hospital setting, the mental health technician may perform routine nursing tasks such as taking pulse, blood pressure and respiration rates. The following are settings in which they work:

- Residential treatment programs
- Psychiatric treatment facilities
- Acute psychiatric units
- Institutes for mental disease
- Psychiatric emergency teams
- State developmental centers
- Long-term care facilities
- Substance abuse programs
- Home health care
- State hospitals
- State prisons
- Intermediate care facilities
- Psychiatric health facilities
- County jails
- Social rehabilitation facilities
- Adult residential facilities
- Secured geriatric facilities
- Day treatment programs
- Outpatient mental health clinics
- Psychiatric assessment centers
- Psychiatric crisis units
- Mobile psychiatric emergency teams
- Special school programs
- Residential care homes
- Partial hospitalization programs

Professional Standards of Practice

Standard 1 – Documentation
The Mental Health Technician systematically and continuously collects data about the health and functional status of clients/patients. This data is recorded, accessible and communicated.

The Mental Health Technician:

1. Informs the client/patient, family and/or significant others of their mutual roles and responsibilities in the data-gathering process.
2. Uses clinical judgment to determine what information is needed. Assessment of health status data includes:
   a. Demographic data:
      (1) Name
      (2) Birth date
      (3) Gender
      (4) Cultural background, religious preference, marital status, and other relevant history.
   b. Baseline data:
      (1)Height
      (2) Weight
      (3) Allergic reactions
      (4) Vital signs
      (5) Hepatitis antigen and antibody status
      (6) Tuberculosis status
      (7) Other relevant nursing history, surgeries, major medical conditions
   c. Medications or treatments of special nursing concern
   d. Seizures: Type and frequency
   e. Pica behavior
   f. General appearance
   g. Mobility status
   h. Hearing and vision status
   i. Prostheses -- Dentures, corrective lens, hearing aid, artificial limb, other adaptive equipment
   j. Physical assessment -- Skin conditions, scalp, teeth, gums, sexual characteristics and development
   k. Patterns in:
      - Nutrition and eating
      - Sleep and rest
      - Elimination
      - Menstruation

3. Functional status data includes:
    a. Level of independent functioning in:
        Toileting
        Dressing
        Hygiene and grooming
        Bathing
        Feeding and Eating
    b. Communication Skills: Language, verbal and non-verbal patterns
    c. Socialization and the level of ability to engage in or initiate:
        Social relationships
        Leisure activities
        Schedule awareness -- appointments, classes, work, etc
    d. Major behavioral concerns affecting health status
    e. Capability for self-administration of medication
    f. Need for sex education
4. Collects data from:
    a. Client/patient
    b. Family
    c. Healthcare personnel
    d. Relevant service providers
5. Collects data by appropriate methods:
    a. Interview and/or observation
    b. Examination
    c. Review of records and reports
    d. Consultation
    e. Collect complete data initially and update information continuously

Standard 2 – Planning
The Mental Health Technician assists in developing a plan with goals and interventions unique to the needs of each client/patient.

The Mental Health Technician:
1. Collaborates with interdisciplinary team members in establishing individualized plans in which:
    a. Priorities of care are identified.
    b. Realistic goals are stated in measurable and observable terms with an expected date of accomplishment.
    c. Goals to maximize functional capabilities are established congruent with:
        (1) Growth and development principles
        (2) Bio-psychosocial principles
        (3) Normalization principles
        (4) Holistic health care principles
    d. Goals are developed for attaining self-help skills, preventing disease, and achieving and maintaining health.
2. Collaborates in the revision of the care plan as goals are achieved or modified

Certified Mental Health Technician

Standard 3 – Intervention

The Mental Health Technician intervenes as guided by the interdisciplinary treatment plan to implement actions that promote, maintain or restore health, prevent illness and promote habilitation.

The Mental Health Technician:
1. Performs interventions consistent with the treatment plan and with competence, efficiency and safety
2. Documents interventions with written records
3. Assists in reviewing the outcome of interventions and making modifications based on progress of the client/patient
4. Interprets interventions to professional and paraprofessional care-givers
5. Ensures that healthcare needs are met by using nursing skills or by obtaining assistance from other healthcare providers
6. Acts as the advocate of the client/patient when necessary to facilitate the achievement of health

Standard 4 – Evaluation

The Mental Health Technician participates in the evaluation of client/patient responses to nursing actions in order to assess progress towards meeting healthcare objectives of the client/patient.

The Mental Health Technician:
1. Uses current data about the client/patient to assist in the measurement of progress toward goal achievement
2. Communicates the degree of goal achievement to the other interdisciplinary team members
3. Assists in the evaluation, shares insights and observations with colleagues and documents the results of the evaluations

Standard 5 -- Interdisciplinary collaboration

The Mental Health Technician functions as an integral member of an interdisciplinary team.

The Mental Health Technician:
1. Is an active participant in setting goals, establishing plans and making decisions
2. Helps ensure that the input of the client/patient is included in this process whenever possible.
3. Respects other clinical discipline members and their contributions to the care of the client/patient
4. Seeks consultation with others when needed and, in turn, provides consultation when appropriate.
5. Gives input and coordinates knowledge and skills with other members of the healthcare team.

Standard 6 -- Peer review

The Mental Health Technician participates in peer review and other means of evaluation to assure quality nursing care.

The Mental Health Technician:
1. Assumes responsibility for review and evaluation of practice with peers
2. Considers recommendations for change that may arise from the review process and implements recommendations

Standard 7 -- Continuing education

The Mental Health Technician assumes responsibility for continuing education and professional development and contributes to the professional growth of others. The scientific, cultural, social and political changes characterizing our society require the Mental Health Technician be committed to the ongoing pursuit of knowledge that will enhance professional growth.

Standard 8 -- Healthcare programs

The Mental Health Technician participates with other members of the community in assessing, planning, implementing and evaluating the community's programs for mental illness and developmental disabilities.

Standard 9 -- Research

The Mental Health Technician contributes to nursing and the mental and developmental health field through innovations in theory and practice, and participation in research.

Required Job-Related Knowledge or Ability

Demonstrating Intervention Techniques
1. Record/report potentially dangerous behavior.
2. Identify behavior that signals an impending crisis, including elopement risk and suicidal or homicidal behavior.
3. Restrain a patient verbally.
4. Restrain a patient physically.
5. Apply restrictive devices to a patient.
6. Demonstrate ways of calming patients.
7. Differentiate between seclusion and "time out."
8. Intervene in patient conflicts.
9. Observe/report/record the level of aggression.

Certified Mental Health Technician

Planning and Administering Patient Care

1. Explain the role of the Mental Health Technician in procedures for individual patient care.
2. Assist in determining appropriate goals for patients.
3. Observe/report progress of individual patients.
4. Provide care in accordance with individual treatment plan.
5. Observe and report changes in patient's physical appearance.
6. Maintain documentation of patient's status, accidents, or unusual behavior.
7. Prepare patient reports as required.
8. Assist in locating missing patients.
9. Report patient comments regarding medication and physical status.
10. Identify signs and symptoms of mental illness.
11. Identify signs and symptoms of physical illness.

Assisting Patients with Rehabilitation

1. Direct structured and unstructured leisure activities.
2. Identify patients' daily schedule of activities.
3. Demonstrate procedures to ensure patient hygiene and personal comfort.
4. Escort patients to and from activities and appointments inside and outside the facility.
5. Maintain safety in patients' living area.
6. Ensure cleanliness in patients' living area.
7. Assist patients in receiving visitors.
8. Assist patients with money management.
9. Assist student-patients with school program.
10. Assist in conducting rehabilitative groups.

Developing Communication and Human Relation Skills

1. Develop rapport with patients.
2. Communicate effectively with patients, staff, and non-facility personnel.
3. Describe therapeutic behavior for effective patient-aide relations.
4. Facilitate interaction among patients.

Fulfilling Environmental and Legal Responsibilities

1. Explain institutional policies and procedures affecting mental health techs.
2. Explain legal policies affecting mental health techs.
3. Ensure continuity of patient information with incoming staff.
4. Search for contraband as directed.
5. Identify methods of assisting patients in exercising their rights.
6. Assist in protecting patients' personal property and valuables.

Certified Mental Health Technician

Psychiatric Disorders

Students should have a good understanding of the following disorders, syndromes and therapies:

Psych Disorders

Schizophrenia
Paranoid Psychotic Disorder
Catatonic Psychotic Disorder
Hallucinations
Bipolar Disorder
Depression
Suicidal Ideation / Attempts
Delusional Disorders
Anxiety Disorders
Panic Attacks
Phobias
Obsessive / Compulsive Disorder
Dissociative Identity Disorder

Personality Disorders

Cluster A - Paranoid / Schizoid
Cluster B - Antisocial / Borderline
Cluster C - Anxious / Fearful

Eating Disorders

Anorexia Nervosa
Bulimia Nervosa
Obesity

Interventions / Therapies

Assist With
Crisis Intervention
Therapeutic Communication
Therapeutic Milieu
Education or Vocational Training
Independent Living Skills
Drug & Alcohol Education
Assaultive Behavior

Assist With Alternative Therapies

Biofeedback
Guided Imagery
Expressive Therapy (Art, Movement)
Massage Therapy
Meditation
Recreational Therapy
Therapeutic Touch
Electro-Convulsive Therapy

Assist With Psychotherapy

Individual
Group
Couple / Family
Behavioral

Additional Disorders

Sexual Disorders
Sexual Abuse / Assault
Survivor of Abuse / Violence
Post Traumatic Stress Disorder
Somatoform Disorders (Pain etc.)
Mental Retardation
ADHD
Developmental / Autistic Disorders

Cognitive Disorders

Delirium
Dementia
Alzheimer's (Dementia)
Amnesic Disorders

Substance-Related Disorders

Alcohol related
Drug Related

Advance Directives

Advanced care directives (i.e., power of attorney; DNR; Do not resuscitate; Living will, etc.) are specific instructions, prepared in advance, that are intended to direct a person's medical care if he or she becomes unable to do so in the future. Advanced care directives allow patients to make their own decisions regarding the care they would prefer to receive if they develop a terminal illness or a life-threatening injury. Advanced care directives can also designate someone the patient trusts to make decisions about medical care, if the patient becomes unable to make (or communicate) these decisions.

Federal law requires hospitals, nursing homes, and other institutions that receive Medicare or Medicaid funds to provide written information regarding advanced care directives to all patients upon admission.

Discharge Planning

For many patients, getting ready to leave the hospital is one of the most critical aspects of their hospital stay. This is truly a critical part of the care and treatment of the patient as inadequate discharge planning can contribute to homelessness among people with serious mental illnesses and/or substance use disorders.

Proper planning for departure from the hospital can make all the difference in patients' long-term prognosis because it encourages them to get involved in managing their own care.

Discharge Planning And Home Follow-Up Of Elders

Http://Www.Guideline.Gov/Summary/Summary.Aspx?Doc_Id=3517

Assessment
- Initiate assessment for discharge planning process at time of admission; continue to reassess throughout hospitalization.
- Focus on those older adults at high risk for poor post discharge outcomes.
- Assessment should include:
    - Functional status (ability to complete instrumental activities of daily living [IADL] and activities of daily living [ADL] and/or functional independence measure [FIM])
    - Cognitive status (ability to participate in discharge planning process and ability to learn new information)
    - Psychological status of patient, particularly depression screening
    - Patient's perception of self-care ability
    - Physical and psychological capabilities of family/caregiver
    - Knowledge deficits regarding health care needs post discharge
    - Environmental factors of post discharge setting
    - Caregiver formal and informal support needs
    - Nine core caregiving processes that ensure family caregivers can provide care smoothly and effectively
    - Review of medications and simplification of regimen
    - Prior link to community services

Implementation of the Discharge Plan

Certified Mental Health Technician

11

- General principles
  - The discharge plan should be tailored to individual patient and family/caregiver needs.
  - Assessment findings will guide intervention strategies.
  - Assessment findings will determine educational and other home health requirements after discharge.
  - Assessment data may predict potential discharge outcomes.
  - Discharge planning should begin at admission due to shortened length of stay and complexities of the population.
  - The discharge plan should be tailored to individual patient and family/caregiver needs.
- Strategies to ensure continuity of care (the 4 Cs: communication, coordination, collaboration, continual reassessment)
  - Communication
    - Communication should occur multi-directionally.
    - Communication should occur between the multidisciplinary team and the patient and family/caregiver.
    - Communication with formal and informal pre-hospital caregivers should be at admission, ongoing, and prior to discharge.
    - Barriers to communication need to be eliminated.
    - Communication of medical care needs to continue between hospital and community medical provider.
    - Written communication
      - Document assessment findings and home care needs on an interdisciplinary record
      - Summarize hospital course, particularly the following:
        - Include actual or potential sequelae
        - Presentation of unusual symptoms or significant change in status since admission
        - Specific symptom management required (i.e., pain post-surgery and effective management)
        - Medication review and difficulties for patient/family
        - Psychosocial adaptation to stress of illness
        - Anticipated outcomes
        - Advanced directive discussions or decisions
    - Verbal communication of health status and discharge plan with:
      - Patient, family and/or caregiver
      - Primary provider who will follow after discharge
      - Multidisciplinary experts
      - Referrals (e.g., home health agency, other providers of care)
  - Coordination of services/case management
    - Case manager or designated team member should coordinate the multidisciplinary team in the discharge planning process.
    - Case manager will link the person with the most appropriate services post discharge.

Certified Mental Health Technician

- Case manager should ascertain understanding of all communication with patient and family/caregiver.
    - Communication should be clear between hospital case manager and home health provider and/or any community resources.
  - Collaboration
    - Multidisciplinary team members should be used for specialized assessments, recommendations, and case conferences.
    - Advanced practice nurse or registered nurse (RN) expert in geriatrics may collaborate with team and provide home follow-up.
    - Designate a case manager or nurse expert in geriatrics to coordinate discharge plan.
    - Family or caregiver can provide information about past experiences, potential barriers, and bio-psychosocial needs of the patient.
    - Referrals should occur in-hospital, when possible, to limit transfers from home environment.
  - Continual reassessment
    - The discharge planning process is dynamic, not static.
    - Status of the patient may change rapidly in this population, requiring frequent reassessment.
    - Change in condition should be communicated to all team members.
    - Home care needs change as the assessment is clarified and as the patient status changes.
- The Discharge Planning Process
  - Develop the plan to meet unique needs of each individual patient and family/caregiver.
  - Communication with pre-hospital formal and informal caregivers should be at admission, ongoing, and prior to discharge.
  - Involve the patient and family throughout discharge planning process.
  - Yield to patient and family wishes and preferences for optimal outcomes.
  - Health teaching, guidance, and counseling (potential areas to address):
    - Gear teaching to specific learning needs of elderly patient.
    - Describe required care related to presenting problem.
    - Describe diet restrictions, and discuss patient preferences.
    - Discuss medication actions and side effects.
    - Discuss symptom management.
    - Define when to call for help.
    - Discuss maintenance of hydration and nutritional status.
    - Delineate signs of a change of condition and whom to report to.
    - Discuss what to report or do in an emergency.
    - Discuss whom to contact in an emergency.
    - Clarify activity level and ability, with a focus on safety and mobility.
    - Discuss and/or clarify advanced directives and care wishes of patient.
    - Verbally review written discharge instructions and follow-up.
  - Treatments and procedures (potential areas to address):
    - Special procedures/care: wound care, tube feedings, hydration etc.
    - Discuss how and when to administer medications.

Certified Mental Health Technician

- Discuss activities of daily living (ADL) interventions: mobility, transfers, gait training.
- Surveillance interventions (potential areas to address):
  - Ensure adequate functional status before discharge or refer for appropriate home care needs.
  - Evaluate system-specific physical assessment related to problems or potential problems.
  - Monitor primary problem and potential sequelae.
  - Functional and cognitive status should be continually monitored.
  - Medication understanding, management capabilities, and side effects
  - Transportation access and availability
  - Family/caregiver abilities evaluated continually
  - Psychosocial issues that may affect transition
- Case management (potential activities of Case Manager)
  - Refer to consultants/providers as needed, preferably while in-hospital.
  - Address questions/concerns from patient, caregiver, and health providers.
  - Provide caregiver with contact numbers of care providers (primary care and home health agency, physical therapy and occupational therapy).
  - Provide follow-up care appointments and contact information.
  - Ascertain access to transportation services.
  - Provide information on other community resources.
  - Assess risk for potential poor discharge outcomes (see Table 16.1 in original guideline document) to ensure appropriate discharge services are utilized.
  - Ensure that caregiver support needs are met.

Textbook Learning Objectives:

Students are encouraged to review the "Mental Health Worker: Psychiatric Aide" (Beverly Marshburn, Kay Cox-Stevens) textbook and insure familiarity with the following items from each chapter:

CHAPTER # 1:
1. Activities of daily living (ADL)
2. Assessment needs
3. Both acute and chronic conditions
4. Identify and diagnose patient needs
5. Identify those patients who need additional supervision
6. Recognize the function of a primary therapist and psychotherapy
7. Recognize the role of social workers, marriage, family and child counselors
8. Recognize the difference between a Registered, Licensed Practical and Licensed Vocational Nurse
9. Identify and Empathize with the qualifications of a successful Mental Health Worker.

CHAPTER #2:
1. Erikson's eight stages of development, including acceptable and normal levels of performance
2. The difference and inter-relationship between the id, the ego and the super-ego.
3. Factors that contribute to the individual's role identification
4. Conditions that lead to successful maturity.

CHAPTER #3:
1. The causes of anxiety
2. The difference between homeostasis and pathological anxiety
3. The function of coping mechanisms
4. The characteristics of an anxiety attack
5. The characteristics of a panic attack
6. Hypochondriasis
7. Phobia, including agoraphobia
8. The signs and symptoms of depression
9. The different treatments for anxiety- both short and long term.

CHAPTER #4:
1. The importance of trust
2. The difference between psychosis and paranoia
3. The meaning of demeanor
4. The variables in a patient's processing
5. The nineteen guidelines in gaining a patient's trust
6. The difference between verbal and nonverbal communication
7. The significance of body language
8. The meaning of metacommunication

9. The significance of transference and counter-transference
10. The signs of suicidal ideation

Certified Mental Health Technician

11. Methods of developing conflict resolution

CHAPTER #5:
1. The importance of and correct technique for hand washing
2. The importance and meaning of Standard Precautions
3. The various patterns of proper body mechanics
4. The Anatomy of the Back
5. Methods of ensuring good body mechanics
6. The correct methods to be applied for fire safety
7. Different fire detection procedures
8. The four classifications of a fire
9. The meaning and application of disaster preparedness
10. The correct application of Cardiopulmonary Resuscitation (CPR)
11. The meaning of code blue
12. The meaning of patient elopement and the appropriate response
13. The regulations and limitations for the use of patient electrical appliances
14. The meaning of and techniques for dealing with contraband
15. The meaning of a body check, and the correct application of the technique
16. The meaning of activity safety and the correct application of the technique.

CHAPTER #6:
1. The importance of patient personal hygiene
2. Monitoring activities of daily living (ADL)
3. Monitoring bowel movements and appropriate techniques for necessary intervention
4. The meaning of vital signs including pulse rate, blood pressure, body temperature and rate of respiration
5. Methods of measuring the pulse
6. Variations in a patient's pulse including the identification of tachycardia and bradycardia
7. The correct method of auscultation of blood pressure
8. Variations in a patient's blood pressure including hypertension and hypotension
9. Methods of measuring temperature
10. Methods of measuring respiration rates and appropriate rates of ventilation
11. The meaning of a neurological check
12. The correct method of measuring a patient's neurological status
13. The correct methods for measuring a patients height and weight
14. The meaning of documentation and its importance
15. Methods of documentation
16. Classes of medication including their use and side effects.

Certified Mental Health Technician

CHAPTER #7

1. The meaning of dependency
2. The meaning of the twelve-step program
3. The signs and symptoms of alcohol abuse
4. The method of testing for breath alcohol
5. The correct method for operating an ALCO SENSOR IV INTOXIMETER
6. The method for identifying the signs and symptoms of alcohol withdrawal
7. The duties of the mental health worker during the patient's withdrawal, including "DAR" charting
8. The difference between alcohol and substance abuse
9. The method of testing for drug use, including a witnessed urine sample
10. The correct method of removing contaminated gloves
11. The correct procedure for ONTRAK, including the interpretation of results and quality control
12. The correct identification of amphetamines
13. The correct identification of the signs and symptoms of amphetamine use
14. The correct identification of the signs and symptoms of amphetamine withdrawal
15. The function of the mental health worker during withdrawal
16. The function of the mental health worker following withdrawal
17. The correct identification of the signs and symptoms of cannabis use
18. The correct identification of the signs and symptoms of cannabis withdrawal
19. The meaning of psychological dependence
20. The function of the mental health worker during withdrawal
21. The function of the mental health worker following withdrawal
22. The correct identification of the signs and symptoms of cocaine use
23. The meaning of euphoria and auditory hallucinations
24. The correct identification of the signs and symptoms of cocaine withdrawal
25. The function of the mental health worker during withdrawal
26. The function of the mental health worker following withdrawal
27. The correct identification of the signs and symptoms of hallucinogen use
28. The difference between perceptual and cognitive changes
29. The correct identification of the signs and symptoms of hallucinogenic withdrawal
30. The function of the metal health worker during withdrawal
31. The function of the mental health worker following withdrawal
32. The correct identification of the signs and symptoms of PCP use
33. The signs and symptoms of PCP withdrawal
34. The correct identification of the signs and symptoms of PCP withdrawal
35. The function of the mental health worker during withdrawal
36. The function of the mental health worker following withdrawal
37. The correct identification of the signs and symptoms of sedative/hypnotics/anxiolytic use
38. The correct identification of the signs and symptoms of sedative/hypnotics/anxiolytic withdrawal
39. The function of the mental health worker during withdrawal
40. The function of the mental health worker following withdrawal

CHAPTER #8:

1. The significance of the DSM-IV
2. The importance of safety for all patients

Certified Mental Health Technician

3. The signs and symptoms of major depression
4. The function of the mental health worker when dealing with a patient with major depression
5. Appropriate treatment of major depression
6. The importance of identifying a self-destructive patient and being capable of rating the symptoms
7. The meaning and implications for constant observation
8. The signs and symptoms of bipolar disorder with an understanding of mania or hypomania
9. The meaning and significance of delusion
10. Appropriate treatment of bipolar disorder
11. The function of the mental health worker in dealing with patients who have major depression or bipolar disorder
12. The signs and symptoms of schizophrenia
13. The function of the mental health worker when dealing with a patient with schizophrenia
14. Appropriate treatment of schizophrenia
15. Understand the significance of auditory hallucination, nihilistic or paranoid thoughts and loose association in terms of the schizophrenic patient
16. The signs and symptoms of borderline personality disorder (BPD)
17. Appropriate treatment of BPD
18. The function of the mental health worker when dealing with a patient with BPD
19. The signs and symptoms of posttraumatic stress disorder
20. Appropriate treatment of posttraumatic stress disorder
21. The signs and symptoms of dissociative identity disorder (DID)
22. The meaning of co-consciousness
23. Appropriate treatment of DID
24. The function of the mental health worker when dealing with DID
25. The signs and symptoms of antisocial disorder (Sociopath)
26. The function of the mental health worker when dealing with antisocial disorder
27. The signs and symptoms of narcissistic personality disorder (NPD)
28. The function of the mental health worker when dealing with NPD
29. The signs and symptoms of adjustment disorder
30. The function of the mental health worker when dealing with adjustment disorder
31. The signs and symptoms of obsessive compulsive disorder
32. The function of the mental health worker when dealing with obsessive compulsive disorder.

CHAPTER #9

1. The signs and symptoms of dyslexia
2. The signs and symptoms of developmental arithmetic disorder
3. The signs and symptoms of developmental expressive writing disorder
4. The signs and symptoms of speech disorders
5. The appropriate treatment and actions for the four developmental disorders
6. The causes, signs and symptoms of attention deficit/hyperactive disorder (ADHD)
7. The characteristics of children, adolescents and adults with ADHD
8. The appropriate treatment of ADHD
9. The signs and symptoms and treatment of childhood-onset and adolescent-onset conduct disorders.
10. The difference between anorexia nervosa and bulimia nervosa
11. The signs and symptoms and treatment of anorexia nervosa
12. The signs and symptoms and treatment of bulimia nervosa
13. The appropriate discipline of children and adults
14. Time-out
15. Benching
16. Room restriction
17. Restraints

CHAPTER # 10

1. The signs and symptoms of Dementia
    a. Memory
    b. Tasks
    c. Language
    d. Orientation
    e. Judgment
    f. Abstract thinking
    g. Misplacing items
    h. Mood
    i. Initiative
2. The signs and symptoms of Alzheimer's disease
3. Factors that influence Alzheimer's disease
4. Stages of Alzheimer's disease
5. The appropriate care settings for Alzheimer's and Dementia patients
6. The appropriate method of a mental health worker to take a health history
7. The appropriate treatment of a patient with dementia
8. The causes of catastrophic reactions
9. The signs and symptoms of abusive behavior
10. The appropriate treatment of abusive behavior
11. Identify the ABC's of problem solving for the patient with dementia
12. The signs and symptoms of patients with sleep disturbances
13. Sundowner syndrome
14. The appropriate drug treatments for dementia
15. Home care for the dementia patient

CHAPTER # 11

1. The causes, signs and characteristics of mental retardation
2. Gestational disorders
3. Environmental disorders
4. Chromosomal disorders
5. The classifications of the mentally retarded
    a. Mild retardation
    b. Moderate retardation
    c. Severe retardation
    d. Profound retardation
6. Specific types of retardation
7. Retardation from Gestational Causes
    a. Toxoplasmosis
    b. Rubella
    c. Environmental causes
    d. Fetal alcohol syndrome
    e. Lead poisoning
    f. Radiation
    g. Pesticides
8. Identify the signs and characteristics of battered children
9. Retardation from Genetic Abnormalities
10. The signs and characteristics of Down syndrome (trisomy 21)
11. The signs and characteristics of Klinefelter's Syndrome (extra X chromosomal disorder)
12. The signs and characteristics of XXX, XXXX, XXXXX syndrome
13. The signs and characteristics of Chi Du Ch at
14. The signs and characteristics of short arm deletion (Chromosome 4)
15. The signs and characteristics of Hurler's Syndrome (a disorder of abnormal metabolism)
16. The signs and characteristics of Lesch-Nyhan syndrome
17. The signs and characteristics of Cornelia de Lange Syndrome
18. The signs and characteristics of Microephalus
19. The signs and characteristics of Hydrocephalus
20. The signs and characteristics of Pheylketonuria (PKU)
21. The signs and characteristics of the Idiot Savant
22. The signs and characteristics of Cerebral Palsy
23. The signs and characteristics of Autism
24. The role of the mental health worker in the treatment and care of the mentally retarded
25. Nutrition
26. Positioning while eating
27. Seizures
28. Behavioral Therapy
29. Self-injurious behavior

CHAPTER #12

1. Identify patient behaviors that may initiate an assault cycle
    a. Self-assault
    b. Assault on others

Certified Mental Health Technician

2. Identify events under the control of the professional staff
3. Identify assault cycle phases
    a. Triggers
    b. Escalation
    c. Crisis
    d. De-escalation
    e. Recovery
    f. Post-crisis depression
4. Identify appropriate treatments for the patient in an assault cycle
    a. Seclusion
    b. Restraint
    c. Unlocked time-out
    d. Locked time-out
5. Narrative notes
6. The mental health worker's role while a patient is in Seclusion and Restraints
7. The correct procedure for the release from restraints
8. The mental health workers responsibilities in the event of patient/employee injury
9. The implementation of a Legal Hold
10. Locked unit
11. 14-day hold
12. 180 day hold
13. The legal responsibilities of temporary conservator ship

CHAPTER #13
1. The correct guidelines for all types of charting
    a. DAR charting
    b. PBATR charting
    c. SOAP charting
    d. Narrative charting
2. Identifying common phrases and words helpful in charting
3. The mental health worker's responsibilities in writing admission notes
4. The mental health worker's responsibilities in writing discharge notes
5. Understanding report and staff assignments
    a. Kardexes
    b. Report sheets
    c. Common chart forms
6. The mental health worker's responsibilities in writing care plans

CHAPTER #14

1. Identify and understand basic patients' rights
2. Identify and understand informed consent
3. Understand the importance and parameters of confidentiality
4. Identify the components and preparation of an incident report
5. The responsibilities of the mental health worker in implementing and maintaining all patient levels
6. Behavioral level
7. Going outside the facility
8. Dealing with families and visitors

Certified Mental Health Technician

Neurology test questions

True/False
Indicate whether the statement is true or false.

_____ 1. A single long extension of the nerve cell body that transmits the nerve impulse away from the cell body is called an axon.

_____ 2. The sympathetic division of the autonomic nervous system stimulates digestion, urination, defecation, and restores or slows down other activities.

_____ 3. Schwann cells are located only in the peripheral nervous system and make up the neurilemma and myelin sheath.

_____ 4. Bipolar neurons have one dendrite and one axon.

_____ 5. The autonomic nervous system uses adrenaline (also called epinephrine) as the transmitting agent.

_____ 6. A deep bridge of nerve fiber known as the corpus callosum connects the two cerebral hemispheres.

_____ 7. The cerebellum is the largest portion of the brain.

_____ 8. The sympathetic division of the autonomic nervous system prepares the body for stressful situations that require energy expenditure, like increasing heart beat and respiratory rate to flee from a threatening situation.

_____ 9. The parasympathetic division of the autonomic nervous system operates under normal nonstressful conditions.

_____ 10. The sclera regulates the amount of light that enters through the pupil.

_____ 11. Tetanus is caused by the introduction of the bacterium *Clostridium tetani* into an open wound.

_____ 12. Otitis media is another name for a middle ear infection, a common occurrence in young children.

_____ 13. Cerebral palsy is a condition caused by inflammation of brain tissue, usually caused by a virus and transmitted by the bite of a mosquito.

_____ 14. Color blindness is an X-chromosome inherited genetic trait occurring more frequently in males, resulting in the inability to perceive one or more colors.

_____ 15. All sensory information is picked up in the central nervous system.

_____ 16. It is the cerebellum that actually allows a person to be aware of sensory stimulation.

_____ 17. Effectors of the nervous system include the lungs.

_____ 18. Neurons are not able to divide.

_____ 19. Membrane potential exists when the membrane is depolarized.

_____ 20. When a neuron is at rest, the outside of its membrane is positively charged.

_____ 21. A nerve impulse is the flow of electrical current along the axon membrane.

_____ 22. A nerve impulse is the flow of electrolytes along and axon membrane.

_____ 23. After an impulse has passed along an axon, the axon returns to the repolarized state.

_____ 24. As long as an axon is repolarized it cannot conduct another impulse.

_____ 25. The tissues of the central nervous system are so delicate that they must be protected by the blood-brain barrier.

_____ 26. The tissues of the central nervous system are so delicate that they must be protected by the foramen magnum.

_____ 27. The central canal of the spinal cord contains blood vessels.

_____ 28. The central canal of the spinal cord contains cerebrospinal fluid.

_____ 29. The cerebral cortex stores memories.

_____ 30.
   the ventricles are cavities found on the surface of the brain.

_____ 31. Vital functions are regulated by the thalamus.

_____ 32. The diencephalon contains the ventricles.

_____ 33. The hypothalamus maintains homeostasis.

_____ 34. The hypothalamus regulates heart rate and blood pressure.

_____ 35. When teaching patients how to avoid brain and spinal cord injuries you will recommend that they completely stop consuming alcohol.

_____ 36. A person is 20% more likely to be brain injured if they bike without a helmet than if they wear one.

_____ 37. The peripheral nervous system is part of the central nervous system.

_____ 38. There are 16 pairs of cranial nerves.

_____ 39. Ganglia are collections of neuron cell bodies.

_____ 40. Most headaches can be treated effectively with over the counter drugs.

_____ 41. Medical treatment should be sought for all headaches.

Multiple Choice
Identify the choice that best completes the statement or answers the question.

_____ 42. The short, branched nerve fibers on the nerve cell that are the receptive areas of the neuron are known as the _____.
   a. dendrites   c. astrocytes
   b. axons   d. tracts

_____ 43. A bundle of nerve fibers located inside the central nervous system is called a(n) _____.
   a. ganglia   c. tract
   b. neuroglia   d. astrocyte

_____ 44. The simplest pathway able to receive a stimulus, enter the central nervous system for immediate interpretation, and produce a response is known as a _____.
   a. nucleus   c. tract
   b. reflex arc   d. synapse

_____ 45. The outermost layer of the meninges (the words meaning "tough mother") is the _____.
   a. dura mater   c. arachnoid mater
   b. pia mater   d. cortex

_____ 46. The middle layer of the meninges, known as the "spider layer," is called the _____.
   a. dura mater   c. arachnoid mater
   b. pia mater   d. cortex

Certified Mental Health Technician

47. The body's control center and communication network, which directs the functions of the body's organs and systems, is (the) ____.
   a. acetylcholine
   b. reflex arc
   c. neuroglia
   d. nervous system

48. An involuntary reaction to an external stimulus is known as a(n) ____.
   a. reflex
   b. action potential
   c. resting potential
   d. reflex arc

49. Star-shaped cells that twine around neurons for support in the brain and spinal cord and connect neurons to blood vessels are known as ____.
   a. microglia
   b. ganglia
   c. astrocytes
   d. axons

50. Small cells that protect the central nervous system by engulfing and destroying microbes and cellular debris are called ____.
   a. horns
   b. neuroglia
   c. astrocytes
   d. microglia

51. Sensory neurons that convey information from receptors in the periphery of the body to the brain and spinal cord are also known as ____.
   a. afferent nerves
   b. efferent nerves
   c. horns
   d. microglia

52. Transmission of nerve impulses across the synapses is brought about by the secretions of very low concentrations of the chemicals known as ____.
   a. neurotransmitters
   b. dopamines
   c. endorphins
   d. chromatids

53. Motor neurons that convey information from the brain and spinal cord to muscles and glands are called ____.
   a. afferent nerves
   b. efferent nerves
   c. horns
   d. microglia

54. Nerve cell bodies located outside the central nervous system are called ____.
   a. microglia
   b. ganglia
   c. astrocytes
   d. axons

55. The three layers of connective tissue membranes that cover and protect the spinal cord and brain are the ____.
   a. Nissl bodies
   b. neurofibral nodes
   c. meninges
   d. ventral roots

56. The area where the terminal branches of an axon are close to, but not touching, the ends of the dendrites of another neuron is called a(n) ____.
   a. synapse
   b. horn
   c. tract
   d. ganglia

57. Neurons that detect stimuli in the environment are known as ____.
   a. synapses
   b. axons
   c. receptors
   d. stimulants

58. The part of the nervous system that consists of the brain and spinal cord is known as the ____.
   a. autonomic nervous system
   b. central nervous system
   c. peripheral nervous system
   d. somatic nervous system

59. The part of the nervous system that consists of all the nerves that connect the brain and spinal cord with sensory receptors, muscles, and glands is known as the ____.
   a. autonomic nervous system
   b. central nervous system
   c. peripheral nervous system
   d. somatic nervous system

60. A bundle of nerve cells or fibers is known as a(n) ____.
   a. root
   c. axon

Certified Mental Health Technician

b. horn   d. nerve

61. Over 60% of all brain cells are ____.
    a. neuroglia cells   c. Nissl bodies
    b. ganglia cells   d. arachnoid cells

62. The cells that are located only in the peripheral nervous system and make up the neurilemma and myelin sheath are the ____.
    a. neuroglia cells   c. Schwann cells
    b. ependymal cells   d. arachnoid cells

63. The cells that form the lining of the cavities in the brain and spinal cord are the ____.
    a. neuroglia cells   c. Schwann cells
    b. ependymal cells   d. arachnoid cells

64. Neurons that have several dendrites and one axon are known as ____.
    a. neurofibral nodes   c. multipolar neurons
    b. unipolar neurons   d. bipolar neurons

65. Gaps in the myelin sheath that allow ions to flow freely from extracellular fluids to the axons are known as ____.
    a. nodes of Ranvier   c. dorsal roots
    b. Schwann cells   d. Nissl bodies

66. Neurons that have one dendrite and one axon are known as ____.
    a. neurofibral nodes   c. multipolar neurons
    b. unipolar neurons   d. bipolar neurons

67. Neurons that have only one process extending from the cell body are known as ____.
    a. neurofibral nodes   c. multipolar neurons
    b. unipolar neurons   d. bipolar neurons

68. Nerve cell bodies that are found outside the central nervous system are generally grouped together to form ____.
    a. ganglia   c. roots
    b. tracts   d. dendrites

69. Areas of gray matter in the spinal cord are called ____.
    a. tracts   c. horns
    b. ependymal cells   d. astrocytes

70. Nerve cells that transmit nerve impulses in the form of electrochemical changes are known as ____.
    a. horns   c. ependymal cells
    b. endorphins   d. neurons

71. The neuroglial cells that form the fatty myelin sheath on the neurons of the brain and spinal cord are the ____.
    a. oligodendroglia   c. microglia
    b. astrocytes   d. ganglia

72. The cells that line the fluid-filled ventricles of the brain are the ____.
    a. glial cells   c. Schwann cells
    b. ependymal cells   d. neurolemmocytes

73. The term that refers to groups of myelinated axons from many neurons supported by neuroglia is ____.
    a. gray matter   c. white matter
    b. horns   d. Nissl bodies

74. The correct number of pairs of cervical nerves is ____.
    a. one (1)   c. twelve (12)
    b. eight (8)   d. five (5)

75. The correct number of pairs of thoracic nerves is ____.
    a. one (1)   c. twelve (12)

Certified Mental Health Technician

b. eight (8)   d. five (5)

76. The correct number of pairs of lumbar nerves is ____.
   a. one (1)   c. twelve (12)
   b. eight (8)   d. five (5)

77. The correct number of pairs of coccygeal nerves is ____.
   a. one (1)   c. twelve (12)
   b. eight (8)   d. five (5)

78. The phrase that means "tough mother" is ____.
   a. pia mater   c. dura mater
   b. arachnoid mater   d. cortex

79. The elevations or folds on the surface of the cerebrum are called ____.
   a. sulci   c. ventricles
   b. gyri   d. tracts

80. The prominent fissure that separates the cerebrum into right and left halves or hemispheres is the ____.
   a. longitudinal fissure   c. corpus callosum
   b. insula   d. transverse fissure

81. The white, outermost layer of the eyeball, composed of tough connective tissue, is the ____.
   a. iris   c. cornea
   b. pupil   d. sclera

82. The area of sharpest vision in the retina of the eye is known as the ____.
   a. pupil   c. fovea centralis
   b. iris   d. optic disk

83. The innermost layer of the eye is called the ____.
   a. pupil   c. aqueous humor
   b. iris   d. retina

84. The area of the retina where the nerve fibers leave the eye is known as the ____.
   a. optic disk   c. iris
   b. pupil   d. fovea centralis

85. The membrane that separates the external ear canal from the middle ear is known as the ____.
   a. tympanic membrane   c. stapes
   b. oval window   d. round window

86. Inflammation of the meninges caused by bacterial or viral infection that results in headache, fever, and a stiff neck is known as ____.
   a. otitis   c. encephalitis
   b. meningitis   d. choroiditis

87. A condition that is a normal part of aging, commonly occurring during the forties, and resulting in a decrease in the ability of the eye to accommodate for near vision is known as ____.
   a. glaucoma   c. presbyopia
   b. myopia   d. cataracts

88. The ability to see close objects but not distant ones is known as ____.
   a. myopia   c. presbyopia
   b. hyperopia   d. glaucoma

89. A disorder in which certain parts of the brain are overactive, producing convulsive seizures and possible loss of consciousness, is ____.
   a. cerebral palsy   c. encephalitis
   b. Parkinson's disease   d. epilepsy

90. An inflammation of brain tissue, usually caused by a virus and transmitted by a mosquito bite, is known as ____.

Certified Mental Health Technician

a. cerebral palsy   c. encephalitis
b. Parkinson's disease   d. epilepsy

_____ 91. A disease characterized by tremors of the hand when resting and a slow, shuffling walk with rigidity of muscular movements is known as _____.
a. cerebral palsy   c. encephalitis
b. Parkinson's disease   d. epilepsy

_____ 92. Elevations of the tongue are called _____.
a. papillae   c. incus
b. gyri   d. sulci

_____ 93. The part of the eye that consists of smooth muscles that hold the lens in place is called the _____.
a. gyri   c. optic tracts
b. ciliary body   d. sulci

_____ 94. The colored part of the eye is the _____.
a. retina   c. cornea
b. pupil   d. iris

_____ 95. Another name for earwax is _____.
a. cerumen   c. sweat
b. sebum   d. rhodopsin

_____ 96. The flexible, visible part of the ear (the ear flap) is called the _____.
a. stapes   c. auricle
b. incus   d. cochlea

_____ 97. The opening in the center of the colored part of the eye, which allows light to enter the eye, is known as the _____.
a. sclera   c. iris
b. pupil   d. cornea

_____ 98. The transparent part of the outermost layer of the eye is the _____.
a. sclera   c. iris
b. pupil   d. cornea

_____ 99. The photo-sensitive cells in the retina that function in dim light, but do not produce color vision, are called the _____.
a. rods   c. ciliary body
b. cones   d. gyri

_____ 100. The photo-sensitive cells in the retina that require lots of light and produce color vision are called the _____.
a. rods   c. ciliary body
b. cones   d. gyri

_____ 101. The cavities within the brain that connect with each other, with the subarachnoid space of the meninges, and with the central canal of the spinal cord are called _____.
a. ventricles   c. gyri
b. sulci   d. fissures

_____ 102. The part of the brain that contains all of the ascending and descending tracts that connect between the spinal cord and various parts of the brain is called the _____.
a. hypothalamus   c. medulla oblongata
b. cerebrum   d. cerebellum

_____ 103. The part of the brain that controls our feelings of rage and aggression, contains the body's thirst center, and maintains waking and sleeping patterns is the _____.
a. cerebellum   c. hypothalamus
b. thalamus   d. cerebrum

____ 104. A condition caused by excessive pressure buildup in the aqueous humor, which can constrict blood vessels entering the eye, is known as ____.
a. glaucoma
c. cataracts
b. conjunctivitis
d. myopia

____ 105. The second layer of the eye, which contains blood vessels and pigment cells, is known as the ____.
a. sclera
c. cornea
b. choroid
d. retina

____ 106. Which of these electrolytes plays and important role in the generation of nerve impulses.
a. calcium
b. potassium
c. phosphate
d. magnesium

____ 107. Anything that inflames the CNS will cause
a. pain
b. the blood-brain barrier to become more permeable
c. motor tremors
d. abnormal respirations

____ 108. The spinal cord ends at which vertebral level?
a. first lumbar
b. first sacral
c. twelfth thoracic
d. coccyx

____ 109. The cervical enlargement of the spinal cord contains
a. a viscous liquid
b. sensory neurons
c. motor neurons
d. muscle fibers

____ 110. A person can consciously inhibit a reflex because
a. the reflex occurs exclusively in the spinal cord
b. all body responses are under voluntary control
c. the impulse goes to the cerebral cortex
d. repolarization occurs in an upward direction.

____ 111. A young woman who has complained of tingling in her fingers and toes is diagnosed with Raynaud's disease. Her doctor has scheduled her for a regional sympathectomy. She asks you what good this will do her. Your best response is
a. You should ask your doctor to explain it to you
b. It will interfere with impulses from nerves that cause blood vessel to constrict.
c. If you don't have is done you may have to have some of your fingers amputated in the future
d. This is a trial surgery. The outcome is not known for sure.

Completion
Complete each statement.

112. _____ or sensory neurons are those that convey information from receptors in the periphery of the body to the brain and spinal cord.

113. A _____ is the simplest pathway able to receive a stimulus, enter the central nervous system for immediate interpretation, and produce a response.

Certified Mental Health Technician

114. Transmission of nerve impulses across synapses is brought about by the secretion of very low concentrations of chemicals called _____ that move across the gap.

115. The short, branched nerve fibers on the nerve cell that are the receptive areas of the neuron are called
_____.

116. _____ or motor neurons are those that convey information from the brain and spinal cord to muscles and glands.

117. The _____ is the middle layer of the meninges.

118. _____ are small cells that protect the central nervous system by engulfing and destroying microbes and cellular debris.

119. Nerve cells are also known as _____.

120. _____ is a condition caused by excessive pressure buildup in the aqueous humor, which can constrict blood vessels entering the eye.

121. The ability of the eye to see distant objects but not close ones is known as farsightedness or
_____.

122. The _____ is the second largest portion of the brain and functions as a reflex center in coordinating complex skeletal muscular movements, maintaining proper body posture, and keeping the body balanced.

123. The _____ is also known as the blind spot of the eye.

124. The posterior part of the eye is filled with _____, which maintains ocular pressure, refracts or bends light, and holds the retina and lens in place.

125. The ear canal is lined with hairs and modified sebaceous glands called _____ glands.

126. The ability to see close objects but not distant ones is known as nearsightedness or _____.

127. A bacterial infection of the conjunctiva of the eye is called _____.

128. Constant stimulation of the semicircular canals of the inner ear due to the motion of a car, boat, or airplane, resulting in nausea and weakness, causes a condition known as _____.

Matching

Match statement with the correct each item below.
a. attach neurons to their blood vessels
b. produce myelin sheath on neurons
c. the middle layer of the meninges
d. nerve cell bodies outside the central nervous system
e. myelinated neurons

____ 129. astrocytes
____ 130. white matter
____ 131. ganglia
____ 132. arachnoid mater
____ 133. oligodendroglia

Match statement with the correct each item below.

Certified Mental Health Technician

a. protective coverings around the brain and spinal cord
b. unmyelinated axons and neuroglia
c. gray matter in the spinal cord
d. engulf and destroy microbes
e. bundles of fibers in the central nervous system

_____ 134. horns
_____ 135. meninges
_____ 136. tract
_____ 137. gray matter
_____ 138. microglia

Match each statement with the correct item below.
a. conveys impulses related to sight
b. controls movements of the eyeball
c. conveys impulses related to smell
d. controls chewing movements
e. conveys impulses related to muscle sense

_____ 139. olfactory nerve
_____ 140. optic nerve
_____ 141. oculomotor nerve
_____ 142. trochlear nerve
_____ 143. trigeminal nerve

Match each statement with the correct item below.
a. transmits impulses related to equilibrium and hearing
b. controls muscles involved in speech and swallowing
c. helps control swallowing and movements of the head
d. controls movements in the pharynx, larynx, and palate
e. controls muscles of facial expression

_____ 144. facial nerve
_____ 145. vagus nerve
_____ 146. accessory nerve
_____ 147. hypoglossal nerve
_____ 148. vestibulocochlear nerve

Match the component of a neuron with its description or function. Answers may be used more than once.
a. cell body
b. axon
c. dendrites
d. Schwann cells

_____ 149. contains mitochondria
_____ 150. produces protein and energy
_____ 151. extend far away from the cell body
_____ 152. send information away from the cell body
_____ 153. branches near the cell body
_____ 154. insulates the axon

Match the classification of neurons to the correct description of each. Answers may be used more than once.
   a. sensory neurons
   b. interneurons
   c. motor neurons

_____ 155. decision makers of the nervous system
_____ 156. afferent neurons
_____ 157. pick up information from receptors at the tips of their dendrites
_____ 158. found only in the central nervous system
_____ 159. efferent neurons
_____ 160. carries impulses to the peripheral nervous system
_____ 161. stimulates glands to secrete

Match these nerve components with the correct description. Answers may be used more than once.
   a. synaptic knob
   b. neurotransmitter
   c. axon diameter

_____ 162. has an effect on the speed of impulse conduction
_____ 163. the end of axon branches
_____ 164. contacts dendrites, cell bodies and axons
_____ 165. cause muscles to contract or relax
_____ 166. cause glands to secrete
_____ 167. inhibits neurons from sending impulses

Match the layers of membranes that cover the CNS, to the correct description. Answers may be used more than once.
   a. meninges
   b. dura mater
   c. pia mater
   d. arachnoid mater
   e. subarachnoid space

_____ 168. toughest layer
_____ 169. all three membrane layers
_____ 170. middle membrane layer
_____ 171. like a spider web
_____ 172. inner most layer
_____ 173. holds blood vessels to the surface of the brain
_____ 174. contains cerebral spinal fluid

The spinal cord is made up of gray matter and white matter. Match the matter to the correct description of it. Answers may be used more than once.
   a. gray
   b. white

_____ 175. inner part of the spinal cord
_____ 176. outer part of the spinal cord
_____ 177. contains neuron cell bodies
_____ 178. contains dendrites

Certified Mental Health Technician

_____ 179. contains myelinated axons
_____ 180. divisions are called horns
_____ 181. divisions are called columns

Match the structure or functions of the spinal cord to the correct descriptions.
a. ascending track
b. descending track
c. reflex arc
d. reflex

_____ 182. carries motor information from the brain to the muscles and glands
_____ 183. carries sensory information to the brain
_____ 184. can cause a motor response without getting information from the brain
_____ 185. an automatic response to a stimuli

Match the parts of the brain with the correct descriptions.
a. cerebrum
b. corpus collosum
c. sulci
d. gyri
e. longitudinal fissure

_____ 186. the groove between the two hemispheres
_____ 187. brain material in between the sulci
_____ 188. largest part of the brain
_____ 189. is divided into two halves
_____ 190. corpus collosum

Match the lobes of the brain to the correct descriptions of their function.
a. frontal
b. parietal
c. temporal
d. occipital

_____ 191. interprets auditory stimuli
_____ 192. interprets visual stimuli
_____ 193. controls motor activity
_____ 194. interprets sensations felt in or on the body

Match these parts of the brain with the corret descriptions.
a. cerebrum
b. brain stem
c. cerebellum
d. pons

_____ 195. connects the cerebrum to the spinal cord
_____ 196. coordinates complex skeletal muscle contractions
_____ 197. located behind the pons and medulla oblongata
_____ 198. is a part of the brain stem
_____ 199. regulates breathing
_____ 200. largest part of the brain

Certified Mental Health Technician

_____ 201. coordinates fine movements

Match these parts of the brain stem with their correct function. Answers may be used more than once.
a. mid brain
b. pons
c. medulla oblongata

_____ 202. controls visual reflexes
_____ 203. has nerve tracks that connect the cerebrum to the cerebellum
_____ 204. controls blood pressure
_____ 205. controls coughing and sneezing reflexes.

Match each cranial nerve to its function. Answers may be used more than once.
a. olfactory
b. trochlear
c. trigeminal
d. facial

_____ 206. innervates muscles for chewing
_____ 207. innervates muscles that move the eyeball
_____ 208. carries sensory information from the tongue
_____ 209. carries smell information to the brain
_____ 210. carries sensory information from the skin of the scalp and face

Match each cranial nerve to its function. Answers may be used more than once.
a. Hypoglossal
b. accessory
c. vagus
d. glossopharyngeal

_____ 211. innervates muscles of the throat, neck and voice box
_____ 212. carries sensory information from the throat
_____ 213. innervates muscles of the tongue
_____ 214. innervates muscles in the stomach, intestines and heart
_____ 215. carries sensory information from thoracic and abdominal regions

Match the two components of the autonomic nervous system to the correct description.
a. sympathetic
b. parasympathetic

_____ 216. releases acetylcholine
_____ 217. slows the heart and respiratory rates
_____ 218. secretes norepinephrine
_____ 219. increases heart rate
_____ 220. activates digestive glands
_____ 221. prepares the body for "flight of fight"

Match the diagnostic test for nervous system disorders with the correct description.
a. lumbar puncture
b. MRI
c. PET scan

Certified Mental Health Technician

d. cerebral angiography

e. electroencephalography

_____ 222. can detect bleeding

_____ 223. can diagnose Alzheimer's and Parkinson's diseases

_____ 224. allows examination of cerebrospinal fluid

_____ 225. detects electrical activity in the rain

_____ 226. useful in detecting aneurysms

_____ 227. useful in diagnosing states of consciousness

Match the types of headaches to their correct description.

a. migraine

b. cluster

c. tension

_____ 228. can occur almost daily for weeks or months

_____ 229. arteries become distended

_____ 230. many are preceded by flashing light or detection of strange odors

_____ 231. most severe and intense of headaches

_____ 232. experienced more often by men

_____ 233. causes soreness in the temples

Match these neurologic disorders with their correct description.

a. Alzheimer's disease

b. amyotrophic lateral sclerosis

c. MS (multiple sclerosis)

d. epilepsy

e. Guillian Barré Syndrome

f. stroke

_____ 234. brain cells die because of a blocked artery

_____ 235. a chronic disease caused by demyelination

_____ 236. the body's immune system attacks the peripheral nervous system

_____ 237. repeated, long term seizure disorder

_____ 238. degenerative disease of the brain

_____ 239. degenerative disease of the spinal cord and brain

Short Answer

240. Place in correct sequence the structures by which an impulse passes through a reflex arc.

a. interneurons

b. sensory neurons

c. motor neurons

d. from receptors

Answer Section

Certified Mental Health Technician

TRUE/FALSE

  1. ANS: T   PTS: 1
  2. ANS: F   PTS: 1
  3. ANS: T   PTS: 1
  4. ANS: T   PTS: 1
  5. ANS: T   PTS: 1
  6. ANS: T   PTS: 1
  7. ANS: F   PTS: 1
  8. ANS: T   PTS: 1
  9. ANS: T   PTS: 1
10. ANS: F   PTS: 1
11. ANS: T   PTS: 1
12. ANS: T   PTS: 1
13. ANS: F   PTS: 1
14. ANS: T   PTS: 1
15. ANS: F
Sensory information is carried by the peripheral nervous system.

PTS: 1
REF: AAMA- Use medical terminology appropriately. Instruct individuals according to their needs.
OBJ: 27-1 | 27-2
16. ANS: F
The cerebral cortex performs that task.

PTS: 1
REF: AAMA- Use medical terminology appropriately. Instruct individuals according to their needs.
OBJ: 27-1 | 27-2 | 27-3
17. ANS: F
The effectors are the muscles and glands.

PTS: 1
REF: AAMA- Use medical terminology appropriately. Instruct individuals according to their needs.
OBJ: 27-1 | 27-2 | 27-3
18. ANS: T   PTS: 1
REF: AAMA- Use medical terminology appropriately. Instruct individuals according to their needs.
OBJ: 27-1 | 27-3
19. ANS: F
Potential exists only when the neuron is polarized.

PTS: 1
REF: AAMA- Use medical terminology appropriately. Instruct individuals according to their needs.
OBJ: 27-5
20. ANS: T   PTS: 1

Certified Mental Health Technician

REF: AAMA- Use medical terminology appropriately. Instruct individuals according to their needs.
OBJ: 27-5

21. ANS: T   PTS: 1
REF: AAMA- Use medical terminology appropriately. Instruct individuals according to their needs.
OBJ: 27-1 | 27-5

22. ANS: F
It is the flow of electrical current.

PTS: 1
REF: AAMA- Use medical terminology appropriately. Instruct individuals according to their needs.
OBJ: 27-1 | 27-5

23. ANS: T   PTS: 1
REF: AAMA- Use medical terminology appropriately. Instruct individuals according to their needs.
OBJ: 27-1 | 27-5

24. ANS: F
That is exactly when it CAN conduct another impulse.

PTS: 1
REF: AAMA- Use medical terminology appropriately. Instruct individuals according to their needs.
OBJ: 27-1 | 27-5

25. ANS: T   PTS: 1
REF: AAMA- Use medical terminology appropriately. Instruct individuals according to their needs.
OBJ: 27-7

26. ANS: F
They are protected by the blood-brain barrier.

PTS: 1
REF: AAMA- Use medical terminology appropriately. Instruct individuals according to their needs.
OBJ: 27-7

27. ANS: F
It contains cerebrospinal fluid.

PTS: 1
REF: AAMA- Use medical terminology appropriately. Instruct individuals according to their needs.
OBJ: 27-9

28. ANS: T   PTS: 1
REF: AAMA- Use medical terminology appropriately. Instruct individuals according to their needs.
OBJ: 27-9

29. ANS: T   PTS: 1
REF: AAMA- Use medical terminology appropriately. Instruct individuals according to their needs.

Certified Mental Health Technician

OBJ: 27-11
30. ANS: F
They are found within the brain.

PTS: 1
REF: AAMA- Use medical terminology appropriately. Instruct individuals according to their needs.
OBJ: 27-11
31. ANS: F
They are regulated by the hypothalamus.

PTS: 1
REF: AAMA- Use medical terminology appropriately. Instruct individuals according to their needs.
OBJ: 27-11
32. ANS: F
It contains the thalamus and hypothalamus.

PTS: 1
REF: AAMA- Use medical terminology appropriately. Instruct individuals according to their needs.
OBJ: 27-11
33. ANS: T   PTS: 1
REF: AAMA- Use medical terminology appropriately. Instruct individuals according to their needs.
OBJ: 27-11
34. ANS: T   PTS: 1
REF: AAMA- Use medical terminology appropriately. Instruct individuals according to their needs.
OBJ: 27-11
35. ANS: F
The emphasis should be to avoid alcohol when engaging in certain activities such as driving or sports.

PTS: 1
REF: AAMA- Use medical terminology appropriately. Instruct individuals according to their needs. Teach methods of health promotion and disease prevention.OBJ: 27-16
36. ANS: F
They are 85% more likely.

PTS: 1
REF: AAMA- Use medical terminology appropriately. Instruct individuals according to their needs. Teach methods of health promotion and disease prevention.OBJ: 27-16
37. ANS: F
It branches off the CNS.

PTS: 1
REF: AAMA- Use medical terminology appropriately. Instruct individuals according to their needs. Teach methods of health promotion and disease prevention.OBJ: 27-12
38. ANS: F

Certified Mental Health Technician

There are 12 pairs.

PTS: 1
REF: AAMA- Use medical terminology appropriately. Instruct individuals according to their needs.
OBJ: 27-14

39. ANS: T   PTS: 1
REF: AAMA- Use medical terminology appropriately. Instruct individuals according to their needs.
OBJ: 27-14

40. ANS: T   PTS: 1
REF: AAMA- Use medical terminology appropriately. Instruct individuals according to their needs. Teach methods of health promotion and disease prevention.OBJ: 27-16

41. ANS: F
Only necessary is headache is chronic.

PTS: 1
REF: AAMA- Use medical terminology appropriately. Instruct individuals according to their needs. Teach methods of health promotion and disease prevention.OBJ: 27-13

MULTIPLE CHOICE

42. ANS: A   PTS: 1
43. ANS: C   PTS: 1
44. ANS: B   PTS: 1
45. ANS: A   PTS: 1
46. ANS: C   PTS: 1
47. ANS: D   PTS: 1
48. ANS: A   PTS: 1
49. ANS: C   PTS: 1
50. ANS: D   PTS: 1
51. ANS: A   PTS: 1
52. ANS: A   PTS: 1
53. ANS: B   PTS: 1
54. ANS: B   PTS: 1
55. ANS: C   PTS: 1
56. ANS: A   PTS: 1
57. ANS: C   PTS: 1
58. ANS: B   PTS: 1
59. ANS: A   PTS: 1
60. ANS: D   PTS: 1
61. ANS: A   PTS: 1
62. ANS: C   PTS: 1
63. ANS: B   PTS: 1
64. ANS: C   PTS: 1
65. ANS: A   PTS: 1
66. ANS: D   PTS: 1
67. ANS: B   PTS: 1

Certified Mental Health Technician

68. ANS: A   PTS: 1
69. ANS: C   PTS: 1
70. ANS: D   PTS: 1
71. ANS: A   PTS: 1
72. ANS: B   PTS: 1
73. ANS: C   PTS: 1
74. ANS: B   PTS: 1
75. ANS: C   PTS: 1
76. ANS: D   PTS: 1
77. ANS: A   PTS: 1
78. ANS: C   PTS: 1
79. ANS: B   PTS: 1
80. ANS: A   PTS: 1
81. ANS: D   PTS: 1
82. ANS: C   PTS: 1
83. ANS: D   PTS: 1
84. ANS: A   PTS: 1
85. ANS: A   PTS: 1
86. ANS: B   PTS: 1
87. ANS: C   PTS: 1
88. ANS: A   PTS: 1
89. ANS: D   PTS: 1
90. ANS: C   PTS: 1
91. ANS: B   PTS: 1
92. ANS: A   PTS: 1
93. ANS: B   PTS: 1
94. ANS: D   PTS: 1
95. ANS: A   PTS: 1
96. ANS: C   PTS: 1
97. ANS: B   PTS: 1
98. ANS: D   PTS: 1
99. ANS: A   PTS: 1
100. ANS: B   PTS: 1
101. ANS: A   PTS: 1
102. ANS: C   PTS: 1
103. ANS: C   PTS: 1
104. ANS: A   PTS: 1
105. ANS: B   PTS: 1
106. ANS: B   PTS: 1
      REF: AAMA- Use medical terminology appropriately. Instruct individuals according to their
      needs.
      OBJ: 27-1 | 27-5
107. ANS: B   PTS: 1
      REF: AAMA- Use medical terminology appropriately. Instruct individuals according to their
      needs.
      OBJ: 27-7
108. ANS: A   PTS: 1

Certified Mental Health Technician

REF: AAMA- Use medical terminology appropriately. Instruct individuals according to their needs.
OBJ: 27-9

109. ANS: C   PTS: 1
REF: AAMA- Use medical terminology appropriately. Instruct individuals according to their needs.
OBJ: 27-9

110. ANS: C   PTS: 1
REF: AAMA- Use medical terminology appropriately. Instruct individuals according to their needs.
OBJ: 27-10

111. ANS: B   PTS: 1
REF: AAMA- Use medical terminology appropriately. Instruct individuals according to their needs. Prepare patient for examinations, procedures and treatments   OBJ: 27-16

COMPLETION

112. ANS: Afferent

PTS: 1
113. ANS: reflex arc

PTS: 1
114. ANS: neurotransmitters

PTS: 1
115. ANS: dendrites

PTS: 1
116. ANS: Efferent

PTS: 1
117. ANS: arachnoid mater

PTS: 1
118. ANS: Microglia

PTS: 1
119. ANS: neurons

PTS: 1
120. ANS: Glaucoma

PTS: 1
121. ANS: hyperopia

PTS: 1
122. ANS: cerebellum

Certified Mental Health Technician

PTS: 1

123. ANS: optic disk

PTS: 1

124. ANS: vitreous humor

PTS: 1

125. ANS: ceruminous

PTS: 1

126. ANS: myopia

PTS: 1

127. ANS: conjunctivitis

PTS: 1

128. ANS: motion sickness

PTS: 1

MATCHING

129.	ANS: A	PTS:	1
130.	ANS: E	PTS:	1
131.	ANS: D	PTS:	1
132.	ANS: C	PTS:	1
133.	ANS: B	PTS:	1
134.	ANS: C	PTS:	1
135.	ANS: A	PTS:	1
136.	ANS: E	PTS:	1
137.	ANS: B	PTS:	1
138.	ANS: D	PTS:	1
139.	ANS: C	PTS:	1
140.	ANS: A	PTS:	1
141.	ANS: B	PTS:	1
142.	ANS: E	PTS:	1
143.	ANS: D	PTS:	1
144.	ANS: E	PTS:	1
145.	ANS: D	PTS:	1
146.	ANS: C	PTS:	1
147.	ANS: B	PTS:	1
148.	ANS: A	PTS:	1
149.	ANS: A	PTS:	1

REF: AAMA- Use medical terminology appropriately. Instruct individuals according to their

Certified Mental Health Technician

needs.

OBJ: 27-1 | 27-4

150. ANS: A   PTS: 1
REF: AAMA- Use medical terminology appropriately. Instruct individuals according to their needs.
OBJ: 27-1 | 27-4

151. ANS: B   PTS: 1
REF: AAMA- Use medical terminology appropriately. Instruct individuals according to their needs.
OBJ: 27-1 | 27-4

152. ANS: B   PTS: 1
REF: AAMA- Use medical terminology appropriately. Instruct individuals according to their needs.
OBJ: 27-1 | 27-4

153. ANS: C   PTS: 1
REF: AAMA- Use medical terminology appropriately. Instruct individuals according to their needs.
OBJ: 27-1 | 27-4

154. ANS: D   PTS: 1
REF: AAMA- Use medical terminology appropriately. Instruct individuals according to their needs.
OBJ: 27-1 | 27-4

155. ANS: B   PTS: 1
REF: AAMA- Use medical terminology appropriately. Instruct individuals according to their needs.
OBJ: 27-4 | 27-5

156. ANS: A   PTS: 1
REF: AAMA- Use medical terminology appropriately. Instruct individuals according to their needs.
OBJ: 27-4 | 27-5

157. ANS: A   PTS: 1
REF: AAMA- Use medical terminology appropriately. Instruct individuals according to their needs.
OBJ: 27-4 | 27-5

158. ANS: B   PTS: 1
REF: AAMA- Use medical terminology appropriately. Instruct individuals according to their needs.
OBJ: 27-4 | 27-5

159. ANS: C   PTS: 1
REF: AAMA- Use medical terminology appropriately. Instruct individuals according to their needs.
OBJ: 27-4 | 27-5

160. ANS: C   PTS: 1
REF: AAMA- Use medical terminology appropriately. Instruct individuals according to their needs.
OBJ: 27-4 | 27-5

161. ANS: C   PTS: 1
REF: AAMA- Use medical terminology appropriately. Instruct individuals according to their needs.

Certified Mental Health Technician

162. ANS: C   PTS: 1
REF: AAMA- Use medical terminology appropriately. Instruct individuals according to their needs.
OBJ: 27-1 | 27-4 | 27-6
163. ANS: A   PTS: 1
REF: AAMA- Use medical terminology appropriately. Instruct individuals according to their needs.
OBJ: 27-1 | 27-4 | 27-6
164. ANS: A   PTS: 1
REF: AAMA- Use medical terminology appropriately. Instruct individuals according to their needs.
OBJ: 27-1 | 27-4 | 27-6
165. ANS: B   PTS: 1
REF: AAMA- Use medical terminology appropriately. Instruct individuals according to their needs.
OBJ: 27-1 | 27-4 | 27-6
166. ANS: B   PTS: 1
REF: AAMA- Use medical terminology appropriately. Instruct individuals according to their needs.
OBJ: 27-1 | 27-4 | 27-6
167. ANS: B   PTS: 1
REF: AAMA- Use medical terminology appropriately. Instruct individuals according to their needs.
OBJ: 27-1 | 27-4 | 27-6

168. ANS: B   PTS: 1
REF: AAMA- Use medical terminology appropriately. Instruct individuals according to their needs.
OBJ: 27-1 | 27-8
169. ANS: A   PTS: 1
REF: AAMA- Use medical terminology appropriately. Instruct individuals according to their needs.
OBJ: 27-1 | 27-8
170. ANS: D   PTS: 1
REF: AAMA- Use medical terminology appropriately. Instruct individuals according to their needs.
OBJ: 27-1 | 27-8
171. ANS: D   PTS: 1
REF: AAMA- Use medical terminology appropriately. Instruct individuals according to their needs.
OBJ: 27-1 | 27-8
172. ANS: C   PTS: 1
REF: AAMA- Use medical terminology appropriately. Instruct individuals according to their needs.
OBJ: 27-1 | 27-8
173. ANS: C   PTS: 1
REF: AAMA- Use medical terminology appropriately. Instruct individuals according to their needs.

Certified Mental Health Technician

OBJ: 27-1 | 27-8
174. ANS: E   PTS: 1
REF: AAMA- Use medical terminology appropriately. Instruct individuals according to their needs.
OBJ: 27-1 | 27-8

175. ANS: A   PTS: 1
REF: AAMA- Use medical terminology appropriately. Instruct individuals according to their needs.
OBJ: 27-9
176. ANS: B   PTS: 1
REF: AAMA- Use medical terminology appropriately. Instruct individuals according to their needs.
OBJ: 27-9
177. ANS: A   PTS: 1
REF: AAMA- Use medical terminology appropriately. Instruct individuals according to their needs.
OBJ: 27-9
178. ANS: A   PTS: 1
REF: AAMA- Use medical terminology appropriately. Instruct individuals according to their needs.
OBJ: 27-9
179. ANS: B   PTS: 1
REF: AAMA- Use medical terminology appropriately. Instruct individuals according to their needs.
OBJ: 27-9
180. ANS: A   PTS: 1
REF: AAMA- Use medical terminology appropriately. Instruct individuals according to their needs.
OBJ: 27-9
181. ANS: B   PTS: 1
REF: AAMA- Use medical terminology appropriately. Instruct individuals according to their needs.
OBJ: 27-9

182. ANS: B   PTS: 1
REF: AAMA- Use medical terminology appropriately. Instruct individuals according to their needs.
OBJ: 27-9 | 27-10
183. ANS: A   PTS: 1
REF: AAMA- Use medical terminology appropriately. Instruct individuals according to their needs.
OBJ: 27-9 | 27-10
184. ANS: C   PTS: 1
REF: AAMA- Use medical terminology appropriately. Instruct individuals according to their needs.
OBJ: 27-9 | 27-10
185. ANS: D   PTS: 1
REF: AAMA- Use medical terminology appropriately. Instruct individuals according to their needs.

Certified Mental Health Technician

OBJ: 27-9 | 27-10

186. ANS: E   PTS: 1
      REF: AAMA- Use medical terminology appropriately. Instruct individuals according to their needs.
      OBJ: 27-1 | 27-11
187. ANS: D   PTS: 1
      REF: AAMA- Use medical terminology appropriately. Instruct individuals according to their needs.
      OBJ: 27-1 | 27-11
188. ANS: A   PTS: 1
      REF: AAMA- Use medical terminology appropriately. Instruct individuals according to their needs.
      OBJ: 27-1 | 27-11
189. ANS: A   PTS: 1
      REF: AAMA- Use medical terminology appropriately. Instruct individuals according to their needs.
      OBJ: 27-1 | 27-11
190. ANS: B   PTS: 1
      REF: AAMA- Use medical terminology appropriately. Instruct individuals according to their needs.
      OBJ: 27-1 | 27-11

191. ANS: C   PTS: 1
      REF: AAMA- Use medical terminology appropriately. Instruct individuals according to their needs.
      OBJ: 27-1 | 27-11
192. ANS: D   PTS: 1
      REF: AAMA- Use medical terminology appropriately. Instruct individuals according to their needs.
      OBJ: 27-1 | 27-11
193. ANS: A   PTS: 1
      REF: AAMA- Use medical terminology appropriately. Instruct individuals according to their needs.
      OBJ: 27-1 | 27-11
194. ANS: B   PTS: 1
      REF: AAMA- Use medical terminology appropriately. Instruct individuals according to their needs.
      OBJ: 27-1 | 27-11

195. ANS: B   PTS: 1
      REF: AAMA- Use medical terminology appropriately. Instruct individuals according to their needs.
      OBJ: 27-1 | 27-11
196. ANS: C   PTS: 1
      REF: AAMA- Use medical terminology appropriately. Instruct individuals according to their needs.
      OBJ: 27-1 | 27-11
197. ANS: C   PTS: 1
      REF: AAMA- Use medical terminology appropriately. Instruct individuals according to their

Certified Mental Health Technician

needs.
OBJ: 27-1 | 27-11

198. ANS: D PTS: 1
REF: AAMA- Use medical terminology appropriately. Instruct individuals according to their needs.
OBJ: 27-1 | 27-11

199. ANS: D PTS: 1
REF: AAMA- Use medical terminology appropriately. Instruct individuals according to their needs.
OBJ: 27-1 | 27-11

200. ANS: A PTS: 1
REF: AAMA- Use medical terminology appropriately. Instruct individuals according to their needs.
OBJ: 27-1 | 27-11

201. ANS: C PTS: 1
REF: AAMA- Use medical terminology appropriately. Instruct individuals according to their needs.
OBJ: 27-1 | 27-11

202. ANS: A PTS: 1
REF: AAMA- Use medical terminology appropriately. Instruct individuals according to their needs.
OBJ: 27-1 | 27-11

203. ANS: B PTS: 1
REF: AAMA- Use medical terminology appropriately. Instruct individuals according to their needs.
OBJ: 27-1 | 27-11

204. ANS: C PTS: 1
REF: AAMA- Use medical terminology appropriately. Instruct individuals according to their needs.
OBJ: 27-1 | 27-11

205. ANS: C PTS: 1
REF: AAMA- Use medical terminology appropriately. Instruct individuals according to their needs.
OBJ: 27-1 | 27-11

206. ANS: C PTS: 1
REF: AAMA- Use medical terminology appropriately. Instruct individuals according to their needs.
OBJ: 27-1 | 27-14

207. ANS: B PTS: 1
REF: AAMA- Use medical terminology appropriately. Instruct individuals according to their needs.
OBJ: 27-1 | 27-14

208. ANS: D PTS: 1
REF: AAMA- Use medical terminology appropriately. Instruct individuals according to their needs.
OBJ: 27-1 | 27-14

209. ANS: A PTS: 1
REF: AAMA- Use medical terminology appropriately. Instruct individuals according to their

needs.
OBJ: 27-1 | 27-14

210. ANS: C   PTS: 1
     REF: AAMA- Use medical terminology appropriately. Instruct individuals according to their
     needs.
     OBJ: 27-1 | 27-14

211. ANS: B   PTS: 1
     REF: AAMA- Use medical terminology appropriately. Instruct individuals according to their
     needs. Teach methods of health promotion and disease prevention.OBJ: 27-1 | 27-14
212. ANS: D   PTS: 1
     REF: AAMA- Use medical terminology appropriately. Instruct individuals according to their
     needs.
     OBJ: 27-1 | 27-14
213. ANS: A   PTS: 1
     REF: AAMA- Use medical terminology appropriately. Instruct individuals according to their
     needs.
     OBJ: 27-1 | 27-14
214. ANS: C   PTS: 1
     REF: AAMA- Use medical terminology appropriately. Instruct individuals according to their
     needs.
     OBJ: 27-1 | 27-14
215. ANS: C   PTS: 1
     REF: AAMA- Use medical terminology appropriately. Instruct individuals according to their
     needs.
     OBJ: 27-1 | 27-14

216. ANS: B   PTS: 1
     REF: AAMA- Use medical terminology appropriately. Instruct individuals according to their
     needs.
     OBJ: 27-13
217. ANS: B   PTS: 1
     REF: AAMA- Use medical terminology appropriately. Instruct individuals according to their
     needs.
     OBJ: 27-13
218. ANS: A   PTS: 1
     REF: AAMA- Use medical terminology appropriately. Instruct individuals according to their
     needs.
     OBJ: 27-13
219. ANS: A   PTS: 1
     REF: AAMA- Use medical terminology appropriately. Instruct individuals according to their
     needs.
     OBJ: 27-13
220. ANS: B   PTS: 1
     REF: AAMA- Use medical terminology appropriately. Instruct individuals according to their
     needs.
     OBJ: 27-13
221. ANS: A   PTS: 1
     REF: AAMA- Use medical terminology appropriately. Instruct individuals according to their
     needs.

Certified Mental Health Technician

OBJ: 27-13

222. ANS: B   PTS: 1
REF: AAMA- Use medical terminology appropriately. Instruct individuals according to their needs. Prepare patient for examinations, procedures, and treatments   OBJ: 27-16
223. ANS: C   PTS: 1
REF: AAMA- Use medical terminology appropriately. Instruct individuals according to their needs. Prepare patient for examinations, procedures, and treatments   OBJ: 27-16
224. ANS: A   PTS: 1
REF: AAMA- Use medical terminology appropriately. Instruct individuals according to their needs. Prepare patient for examinations, procedures, and treatments   OBJ: 27-16
225. ANS: E   PTS: 1
REF: AAMA- Use medical terminology appropriately. Instruct individuals according to their needs. Prepare patient for examinations, procedures, and treatments   OBJ: 27-16
226. ANS: D   PTS: 1
REF: AAMA- Use medical terminology appropriately. Instruct individuals according to their needs. Prepare patient for examinations, procedures, and treatments   OBJ: 27-16
227. ANS: D   PTS: 1
REF: AAMA- Use medical terminology appropriately. Instruct individuals according to their needs. Prepare patient for examinations, procedures, and treatments   OBJ: 27-16

228. ANS: C   PTS: 1
REF: AAMA- Use medical terminology appropriately. Instruct individuals according to their needs.
OBJ: 27-16
229. ANS: A   PTS: 1
REF: AAMA- Use medical terminology appropriately. Instruct individuals according to their needs. Prepare patient for examinations, procedures, and treatments   OBJ: 27-16
230. ANS: A   PTS: 1
REF: AAMA- Use medical terminology appropriately. Instruct individuals according to their needs. Prepare patient for examinations, procedures, and treatments   OBJ: 27-16
231. ANS: B   PTS: 1
REF: AAMA- Use medical terminology appropriately. Instruct individuals according to their needs. Prepare patient for examinations, procedures, and treatments   OBJ: 27-16
232. ANS: B   PTS: 1
REF: AAMA- Use medical terminology appropriately. Instruct individuals according to their needs. Prepare patient for examinations, procedures, and treatments   OBJ: 27-16
233. ANS: C   PTS: 1
REF: AAMA- Use medical terminology appropriately. Instruct individuals according to their needs. Prepare patient for examinations, procedures, and treatments   OBJ: 27-16

234. ANS: F   PTS: 1
REF: AAMA- Use medical terminology appropriately. Instruct individuals according to their needs.
OBJ: 27-16
235. ANS: C   PTS: 1
REF: AAMA- Use medical terminology appropriately. Instruct individuals according to their needs. Prepare patient for examinations, procedures, and treatments   OBJ: 27-16
236. ANS: E   PTS: 1
REF: AAMA- Use medical terminology appropriately. Instruct individuals according to their

Certified Mental Health Technician

needs. Prepare patient for examinations, procedures, and treatments   OBJ: 27-16

237. ANS: D   PTS: 1
    REF: AAMA- Use medical terminology appropriately. Instruct individuals according to their needs. Prepare patient for examinations, procedures, and treatments   OBJ: 27-16

238. ANS: A   PTS: 1
    REF: AAMA- Use medical terminology appropriately. Instruct individuals according to their needs. Prepare patient for examinations, procedures, and treatments   OBJ: 27-16

239. ANS: B   PTS: 1
    REF: AAMA- Use medical terminology appropriately. Instruct individuals according to their needs. Prepare patient for examinations, procedures, and treatments   OBJ: 27-16

SHORT ANSWER

240. ANS:
    1. d
    2. b
    3. d
    4. a

    PTS: 1
    REF: AAMA- Use medical terminology appropriately. Instruct individuals according to their needs.
    OBJ: 27-10

www.ingramcontent.com/pod-product-compliance
Lightning Source LLC
Chambersburg PA
CBHW040747200526
45159CB00023B/1757